Table of Contents

Introduction

Colon hydrotherapy is a process that many people may have never heard about in the past and so they may not understand all that well. For those who have heard of the process, it might sound uncomfortable and they would never want to try it. But as this book shows, it is a great process that can make you feel so much better as well as helping with your digestion and the absorption of the nutrients that you take into your body. This guidebook will help you to understand a bit more about this process, how it can benefit you, and why you should consider having it in your life.

Chapter 1 will take some time to look at the digestive system and how it all works. This is the crucial thing that you will need to understand in order to learn how the colon hydrotherapy is going to be able to assist you. This chapter will spend some time on the different organs, processes, and even hormones that are involved in the whole process of eating so that you are able to get in the nutrients that the body needs from the foods that you are taking in.

Chapter 2 then talks a bit about nutrition and digestion and how it can all help you out. If you are eating a diet that is high in fats and other bad things, like the typical American diet, you are not feeding your body what it needs and this can end up slowing your digestion system down and making you feel horrible. There are also some diets and detoxes that you can try out for when you are trying to switch off the bad diet you have been on and you would like a quick fresh start with it.

Chapter 3 gets into the meat of what colon hydrotherapy is all about. It briefly talks about how this process is going to work and some of the reasons why you might want to consider using this therapy in your life. There are a lot of benefits that come with using this therapy and these will also be discussed in this chapter. Chapter 4 is then going to go into more details about this whole process. You will learn some of the things that you will need to do in order to prepare yourself for the therapy so that you are as relaxed and prepared as possible so the therapy can go better.

Then there will be a general walk through of the whole process so that you will know what to expect when you go in for this therapy rather than being surprised. It is surprisingly easy and other than the wait time for the therapy to do its job, there is not even much time with the whole process at all.

Use this guidebook to start to understand a bit more about this kind of therapy and how it can make a big difference to your life and your overall health. It is a great therapy to use, even though a lot of people may not understand how it is all going to work. After using this book, it will make a lot more sense and you may want to consider it for your own life for much better health.

Chapter 1: The Digestive System and How it Works

Before we take a look at how colon hydrotherapy works, we need to first understand how the digestive system works so that the therapy makes sense for how it can help us out. There are only a few things in the world that are very vital to our being and the digestive system is one of these. Without this system, there is no way that we would be able to get the benefits of the food you eat and soon you will be starving yourself to death.

The digestive system is really vital to your health and well-being. It is the system that will be in charge of first absorbing and then transporting the nutrients that you get from food into the blood so they can be moved to the organs that need them the most. Once that is done, it is the system that is in charge of removing any waste that the body will not be using. It consists of many different parts, but all of them need to be working together in order to get the job done.

To start with, this system is going to be composed of several hollow passageways, starting up at the mouth where you take the food in and then ending down at the anus. These organs are going to be aided with some of your other organs, such as the pancreas and the liver to help get the process done.

The second that you eat some food or drink something, it is going to take a journey throughout the whole body. The journey is much longer than you would think to begin with; when you take out the digestive system from a human body, you will find that it is able to stretch out to being 30 feet, although most of this is going to be the intestines. The food will also take a bit of time to get through this long system as it will usually take a few hours to get it all done. In some cases, issues will arise and it can take even longer to finish, one of the reasons why colon hydrotherapy might be for you.

The best way to understand completely how this system is going to work is to follow some food through it. Take a bite of your sandwich for lunch and let's see where it all goes! Before you even get a bite of the sandwich, the nose is going to pick up some of the smells that come from the food and this will signal the brain to get ready to eat. The brain next works in order to get the mouth to water to help with breaking down the food for easier digestion once it gets to the stomach. Take a bite and let the salivary glands get to work!

When you take a swallow of the sandwich, the pieces are going to go down into the throat or the pharynx where they are going to hit a fork where the trachea for breathing is going to meet up with the esophagus. For the most part, you are going to see that the food will go down the right path into the stomach, but in some cases the food will go down the wrong pipe and you will need to cough it back up or get some help right away so that you are able to breathe. In most cases though, the epiglottis is going to be closed just by you swallowing so the food is only going to have one opening to go down. It will make its way down thanks to some of the muscles that are in the throat and soon it will be past the esophagus and into the stomach.

Now that the food has made it to the stomach, it is going to be prepared for the small intestine for easier absorption. Glands that are inside the stomach will secrete some acid, mucous, and enzymes that will coat the stomach to be safe will also cover the food to get it ready. The smooth muscles of the stomach are going to work to contract every 20 seconds so that the enzymes and acid can work to turn the bite of sandwich into liquid. The amount of time that it takes to digest a food will vary. Sandwiches only take about 20 minutes while other foods could take over an hour and still not be done.

The sandwich is going to continue on the journey in order to get to the beginning of the small intestine. The breaking down process is not done by this point as some enzymes from the pancreas are going to join in as well as the bile from your liver. These juices are going to be mixed in so that the sandwich is ready to move into the jejunum next as well as the ileum. Both of these sections are going to work in order to absorb the water and other nutrients that come from the food before it gets pushed on to the large intestine.

Once all of the good nutrients and water have been taken out of the food, the parts that cannot be digested by the small intestines are going to move on to the large intestine, which is the final part of this process. This intestine is going to try and get some of the extra fluid that is there in order to produce the feces that you will excrete later. The colon is going to use some more involuntary movements to get this waste out. This is going to take some time since it is much slower and the waste will only move about a centimeter each hour.

There are three parts to the large intestine. The first part is the cecum and then the colon. These first two are good at removing fluids and salts from the food once they get to this part. There are millions of bacteria inside the large intestine that will work to ferment and then absorb the other substances that are in the food such as the fiber. They are going to also be able to produce the mucous that is needed to move the feces through the colon easier before it enters the third part of this intestine known as the rectum. In this process, once it gets this far, the feces is going to be excreted through the anus in the next bowel movement.

For the other side of things, the pee is going to be created by the water that was taken out of the food in the small intestine as well as the waste that the cells and other body organs are giving to you when they are done with using the nutrients from the food. This will combine inside the kidneys where they will be excreted the next time that you go to the bathroom.

While the above is the basics that come along with this process, there are a lot of other parts that make the whole digestive system possible for you. Without these other parts, you might find that you are not able to get the nutrients into your body, no matter how much you eat, and you could end up really sick. This section will look at some of the glands, hormones, and organs that are used to keep your digestive system working well.

Organs

The organ that is most helpful to the process of digestion, other than the stomach and intestines of course, is the liver. This is a huge organ that can take up about 2.5 percent of the human body because it has so many jobs to do when it comes to keeping you happy and healthy. When it comes to digestion, the liver is involved in producing and releasing bile, a fluid that is placed into the small intestines by the liver in order to break up, digest, and absorb any fats that come into your stomach. The liver is able to make more bile than it needs at a time so that it is ready to go once you take in some more food. The extra bile will be stored within the gallbladder. When the food you eat starts to go to the intestines, there will be a signal sent to the gallbladder that tells it to give out some bile. In some cases, the gallbladder is going to need to be removed, but this does not mean that you will not be able to digest again. It just means that the liver will store the bile inside its bile ducts instead.

Another organ that is important in helping out with this digestive system is the pancreas. It is smaller compared to the liver, but it is even more efficient at the job it has to do. It works to create juices that are full of enzymes to be used during digestion. The enzymes are able to work to change the chemical component of the food you eat so that it can break down the carbs, fats, and proteins inside the stomach for better absorption.

Glands

You are going to be able to find glands all throughout the digestive system whether it is from the mouth or from the intestines. To start with is the mouth. In this area, the salivary glands are going to start working before you even take a bite of food. The saliva is going to work in order to moisten up the food and it can even break down the starches in the food so they are easier on the stomach when it gets that far.

Once the food gets down to the stomach, the stomach is going to have glands that work to excrete juices that are strong enough to break down the food even more. There are then even more of these once you get to the intestines that are able to further break up the food that you have been eating better than before. These glands are basically responsible for breaking down the nutrients that are in your food so that you are able to get it absorbed and into the body as efficiently as possible.

Hormones

The hormones in your body probably spend the most time helping out the digestive system compared to all of the other parts of this system. The hormones are in control of regulating the whole of the digestive system and some of them can even regulate how hungry or full you feel. There are three hormones that are known for helping out the most when it comes to you eating that sandwich at lunch. These include:

- Gastrin—this is the hormone that is going to send out a signal to the stomach so that it is able to start producing the acid needed in digestion. It is also going to play a big role in the stomach, colon, and small intestine lining growing so that they are able to absorb the nutrients from the food you are eating while also excreting digestive juices.

- Secretin—this is the hormone that is going to communicate with all of the accessory organs of the digestive system. When it goes to the pancreas, this organ is going to start excreting the juices needed for digestion. When it goes to the stomach, this organ is going to start producing pepsin which is used to digest the protein you consume. When it calls to the liver, that organ is going to start producing the bile that is needed for digestion. Without this hormone, it would be very hard to digest the nutrients that your body needs to survive.

- CCK—this is the hormone that is going to talk to the smaller organs that will still be needed in order to help out with digestion such as the gallbladder and the pancreas. This hormone is going to tell the pancreas to grow so that it is able to produce more of the enzymes necessary to aid in digestion. The gallbladder will be waiting for the orders from CCK in order to release any bile that is being stored there from the liver so that it can help as well.

While those are some of the biggest hormones that help out with the digestion process, they are not the only ones to watch for when you want to get a healthy digestion. Another one you might enjoy for this proper digestion is ghrelin. This is a hormone that is produced through the small intestine and the stomach when food is not present inside. When the levels or this hormone are running high, you are going to feel hungry and want to eat. Peptide YY is another hormone that you will find useful and it is used in the opposite way of ghrelin. When there is a lot of this hormone in the body, it is going to make you stop eating because you are not feeling hungry any longer.

The digestive system is a complex system that needs a lot of different parts to work together and to work correctly in order to give you the benefits that you are looking for. If one part is not doing its job, you will find that the whole digestive system is not going to be working as efficiently as before. But when they are all working together and doing the job they have been assigned, you will find that you are able to properly nourish your body and excrete any of the waste that has been made.

Chapter 2: Nutrition and Digestion

One of the first things that you should do when you see there is a problem with your digestive system is to make sure that you are eating the right kinds of foods. None of the other therapies are going to be as effective if you are still eating a lot of unhealthy and processed foods in the diet rather than eating something that is healthy and good for you. So the moment you feel like your digestion is not the best, take a step back and examine the diet that you are eating.

Processed, fast, and sugary foods are going to do horrible things to your digestion. They are going to mess the chemicals that are coming in your stomach so that the digestion is not going to work very well. Plus these foods do not have the nutrition that your body needs so you are digesting a bunch of junk. It is much better to look at some of the better ways of eating so that you are able to get the most out of the food you eat. Sometimes all that you need is a proper detox as well as a good diet in order to get everything lined up just right again. This chapter will explore some of the things that you should consider when it comes to nutrition and digestion in order to keep your system running well.

Eating Clean

The first thing that you should do in order to keep your system running properly is learn how to eat clean. Clean eating is not a hard thing to do, but it is going to take a bit of dedication so that you are able to give up the bad foods and just eat the things that are good for your body. This kind of eating is not going to be just about eating the right foods but also about making sure that you are not eating the processed and junk foods that are so easy to find all over the place.

Some of the principles that come with clean eating so that you can keep yourself and your digestive system running healthy include:

- Eating whole foods—it is best to choose the foods that are as whole and pure as possible. You do not want to pick ones that have fifty ingredients, including ones you cannot pronounce, because these have been so processed in the factory that they are not really food any more. Most of the foods that you will need to eat on this diet are the ones that you could find right out of your garden or on a farm. They would include options like seeds, nuts, dairy products that are low in fat, free range and grass fed meats, vegetables, fruits, and whole grains. These have as few ingredients as possible and so are full of nutrition that your body needs to be healthy and happy.

- Avoid the processed foods—this is basically any foods that have labels on them because this means that there is going to be more than a single ingredient that was used in order to make the food. Of course, you do not have to get rid of all the packaged foods, this would be almost impossible unless you live on a farm and things like natural cheeses and whole grain pastas are fine. But you should make sure to read the labels of the food you would like to eat and see if you are able to pronounce the ingredients. If there are a lot of ingredients that are not recognizable, do not eat this food.

- Avoid the refined sugar—this ingredient is only adding calories to your body and is not going to provide you with any nutritional value. Plus it can spike up your blood sugars to make diabetes a possibility which will make even more issues for your digestive system. There are a few other sweeteners that can be used for your foods, but you will still need to use these with moderation when eating clean.

- Eat small meals—with clean eating, it is believed that eating more meals throughout the day that are smaller is better for your metabolism as well as to keep the cravings at bay. This diet recommends that you eat five to six small meals or snacks each day. This can help you to eat less because you are not going to feel as hungry and you are less likely to splurge on some foods that are just not that good for you.

- Cook at home—it is easy to go out to eat and get some of the meals that you need. But none of the foods that you will be able to get at the fast food restaurant are going to be good for you on a clean eating diet. Make sure to cook your own meals at home so that you are getting ones that are healthy and full of all the good ingredients that your body needs to stay healthy.

- Combine the carbs and the proteins—when you eat your meals or snacks, have them be as balanced as possible. For the best in satisfaction and to avoid the temptation to eat some junk food, you should combine carbs with either a fat or a protein. This will make it easier to get rid of the hunger pangs that you may be dealing with.

Eating this kind of diet is going to help you to get the good food and nutrients that you need in order to keep the digestive system working at its best for a long time to come. It is one of the first things that is going to be required before you are able to do any of the therapies, even if you are not going to do a detox. Keep up with this healthy diet for all of the good benefits, including the good digestion, feeling better, and losing weight.

Juicing

Juicing is a diet form that has been gaining in popularity due to how many great nutrients and vitamins that you are able to get from the fruits and vegetables that you are consuming. Juicing is something that everyone can do because everyone needs more fruits and vegetables added in to their diets every day.

There are many different ways that you can choose to juice. Some people choose to just have a juice on an occasion with a friend and will use one of the many juice bars that have sprouted up over the years. Some people choose to go on juicing diets where they will receive the majority of their calories from juicing in order to lose a lot of weight quickly. And still others will choose to just juice every once in a while when they want a light meal to enjoy or need to get more fruits into their diets.

Many people worry that juicing is going to be expensive for them to follow. If you are choosing to go to a juicing bar every day in order to get your juice, then this whole process can quickly get really expensive. You can easily start juicing from your home and it will not cost much more than the expense of the fruits and vegetables that you choose. Juicing can be a quick and easy process that you can do at anytime and anywhere that you choose.

There are many reasons why people will choose to add juicing into their daily lives. Juicing provides a safe and effective way to get a lot of quality nutrition into your body. There are three reasons why most people cite that juicing is so beneficial to the health. These main reasons include:

- There is very little digestion in juicing so your body can quickly digest the nutrients that it is taking in.

- You can consume more vegetables and fruits through juicing than you would be able to eat. This means that you are able to get more nutrients into your body than you would be able to otherwise.

- Juicing can help you to detox your liver.

In addition to these benefits, there are many benefits that you can experience for your health. To start with, when you juice you will be able to improve both your heart health and your cardiovascular system. The vitamins E and C help to prevent any damages that free radicals will cause to your artery walks along with preventing blood from clotting or sticking. In addition, magnesium and potassium are really important to keep your heart functioning like it is supposed to. Also, when you lose weight through a juicing diet, you will be lowering your risk of heart disease. All of these things added together can make it easier for you to have a really great heart health.

Another health benefit that you can get from juicing is a detox of the liver. Your liver has a lot of functions in your body including removing metabolic waste and toxins and cleaning out your blood. There are certain nutrients that you can consume that will help benefit the liver so that it can keep up with its job. Some good antioxidants that you can consume to get these benefits include beta carotene, vitamin, E, vitamin, C, and several different vitamins B.

Vegetable juices are great if you need to alkalize your system. Fruits will not be able to help you out with this because most fruits will be acidic. There are many benefits to alkalizing your system. Some of these benefits include better digestion, less likely to get sick, better functioning of your joints, ability to slow down your aging process, improved function of the heart, and improved function of the brain.

Drinking plenty of juices can help keep your eyes, nails, hair, and skin healthy as well. There are so many great vitamins that are found in the different juices you can make, especially if you are able to mix and match them up, that you can take care of all these important health issues simply by juicing.

If you have been feeling a little down and like you do not have the energy to do the things that you should be able to during the day, then juicing may be the solution for you. The more that you juice, the more minerals and vitamins that you will get into your system. These vitamins can help you receive the energy that you need to stay healthy all day long

Juicing can even help you to rebuild your blood cells. You will need to make sure to consume some juices that contain dark greens so that you get the chlorophyll that your blood cells need. If you consume enough of this nutrient, your blood cells will start to build up again and you will feel more energized and healthy all over again.

Everyone needs to improve their immune system, especially during the winter months. Drinking some healthy juicing recipes will help you to receive the vitamins and antioxidants that your body needs in order to maintain a good immune system.

Cleanses

The idea behind doing a cleanse is that you want to be able to clean out the body, especially the colon of all the different toxins that have built up there due to your poor diet and lifestyle. When these toxins build up, it is really hard to digest the foods that you are taking in and often it will contribute more to you losing weight.

The best cleanse to try out for your colon is known as the Four Elements Cleanse. Each of these will be talked about more below:

Element One: The Diet

The diet that you are eating is going to be one of the first things that you will need to figure out when you are on a colon cleanse. You will need to eat healthy and whole foods, ones that are full of nutrients that are good for your body rather than ones that can cause it harm and make it bloat up. For example, you should make sure that you are eating foods such as eggs, whole grains, lean meats, vegetables, and fruits. Staying away from sugars and other processed foods is imperative if you are looking to see some great results during this cleanse.

Element Two: The Drinks

The drinks that you should be having during a cleanse will need to be able to help out rather than hinder the progress you are making. This means to drink plenty of water and healthy teas while avoiding other bad things like sodas and coffee. There are also many special drinks, such as the juices mentioned above, that can be used in order to help you to clean out the colon even more. Getting rid of all of the food that might be stuck there and causing issues with your body is a good way to get started before considering any other treatments.

Element Three: Fiber

Often the easiest way to get the colon all cleaned out is to make sure that you are getting in enough fiber. Fiber is going to stick to the sides of the intestines while it slides through, making sure it takes everything it touches along with it. Most people do not get enough food foods into their diet and this can mean they are going to be low on the fiber count that they need. Make sure that you are getting a lot of fiber into your diet each day which should be easier if you are doing the diet that is needed for a colon cleanse, and take a supplement to help out if needed.

Element Four: Take Probiotics

These nutrients are able to help you get a healthy digestive system. These are going to help you in three different ways including boosting your immune system, regulating how much acidity is I the gut, and being able to crowd out pathogens. It is a good idea to take these probiotics on a regular basis if you want to keep the digestive system running strong. There are various supplements that are available or eating some yogurt each day can help you out as well.

The whole point of doing a cleanse is because you think the digestive system is not doing its best, usually because of some other issue that is going on, and you want to help it get all cleared out. When you eat the right foods and drinks and ensure that you are giving the body the nutrients it needs, you are not going to have to worry about this. The cleanse is going to clear out any of the bad stuff that is inside the digestive tract, particularly in the colon, and help to make it all better so that you are able to have the best health.

Detoxing

Detoxes have gained a lot of popularity with a lot of people because it is not only able to clean out the digestive system, but it can clean out a lot of other parts of the body as well. Each of the detox plans you can choose to go with will have different requirements of what you are able to eat and what you need to avoid. Some will want to you fast during them and others are just going to allow you to drink liquids. Even others will allow a few types of foods as long as you pick ones that are healthy and fresh like plenty of fruits and vegetables. Each of them are going to restrict the amount of things that you are allowed to eat in the hopes that the body will be able to clean itself out.

These are going to be higher effort levels compared to the cleanses and other diets that were discussed in this guidebook. You might notice that you are feeling hungry as well as weak. The good news is that you usually will not be on a detox, at least the most restrictive ones that only allow you to have juice, for very long. This is because if you stay on this kind of detox for a long period of time, you will find that you are not getting the nutrients you need in order to stay healthy, you will have nausea, fatigue, muscle aches, low blood sugars, and low energy. None of these are going to make you feel very good and if you go on these for too long, you are going to find that you do not like the diet and will not be likely to stay on it without cheating for much longer.

For some people, the detox for more than a few days is going to be too long and they will not be able to stay on it very well. You might find that trying out a clean eating diet before will help or to use this after you are done with the detox. These clean eating diets are much healthier and can clean out the body as well with all the healthy foods that you are eating. Eating a clean diet detox is better for the long term and can give you a lot of great results. Basically it is going to be required for you to eat foods that are whole and fresh with as few ingredients as possible to feel and look your very best.

The whole point of going on a detox, whether it is about going on a fast or limited one or going on one that just contains the healthier foods that are good for you, is to clean out the body of all the different toxins that are inside. These toxins are often going to make your body weary and it is hard to get the nutrition that you need. When you go into a detox, you are helping the body to flush all of these toxins out so that you can feel your very best.

Going on the proper diet is often one of the best things that you can do in order to make your whole body feel amazing. Before you go with any other treatment options, it is a good idea to try out one of the cleansing options that were listed above. These are often going to be a good way to clear out the body and to make sure that you are not going to leave any toxins inside. Often this is going to be enough for you to clear out the body so that the colon is healthy and can do its job properly.

Chapter 3: What is Colon Hydrotherapy

To understand more about colon hydrotherapy, it is important to understand about how colon cleansing is going to work. All of the different options for nutrition that are listed in the previous chapter are meant to show that you are able to clean out the colon with some more natural means such as with the foods that you are consuming. You do not have to do anything that is crazy or which even needs to use some therapy because often the food and drinks that you are taking in will often be able to determine how well your body is going to digest things and stay healthy.

Colon hydrotherapy is a more specific kind of the colon cleansing that you might consider to stay healthy. This colon cleansing is going to encompass a larger number of medical therapies, all of which claim that they are able to remove some toxins from your body, more specifically from the colon and the rest of the digestive system. Colon cleansing has many different names but it will all mean the same thing of cleaning out the colon.

There are different ways that you can use colon therapies in order to clean out your body. Some will use some tubes in order to inject some water or other liquid into the colon in order to get it all cleaned out for you. Other options will use laxatives, dietary supplements, herbs, and dietary fiber in order to clean out the body and make you feel better when you are done. Of course, you should use some of these in moderation; for example, if you are taking too much of a laxative, you can end up taking it too much and become sick when the nutrients are all gone from your body.

So let's take a look at what colon hydrotherapy is all about. This is a type of treatment that is meant to help out with a large amount of health problems that might include fatigue, intestinal parasites, bowel obstruction, and addiction. Though it is a treatment that is used a lot for many patients, it is important that you take the time to talk to your doctor and ensure that this is going to be safe for you to try before you get started.

Waste product and the bacteria that thrive on them are able to build up in the intestines when they are not taken care of in the proper way. Those who practice colon hydrotherapy will believe that these bacteria are able to cause a lot of different diseases and health issues in the individual who is not able to get them out of the body. They believe that using this kind of therapy is able to clean out the intestines so that the toxins will leave the body. When this therapy is used in the proper way, you will be able to prevent illness and disease, improve the way that your mind is functioning (perhaps due to the fact that it becomes easier to absorb the good nutrients that your body is using), and to affect the immune system in a positive way.

While there are a lot of good things that can happen when you use colon hydrotherapy, it is still important to understand how the process works to help you to determine if it is able to work the best for you. This type of therapy is going to work similar to an enema. What this means is that water will be used during the therapy in order to flush out the bowels. There are some variables that will be used with this process which means that each session of hydrotherapy is going to chance depending on the patient and the goals they have in mind. For example, the water can be used in varying amounts and the pressure and temperatures will be changed depending on why the treatment is being used. In some cases, probiotics, herbs, enzymes, and coffee can be added to the treatment in order to add to the effectiveness to the procedure.

When you go into the treatment, you will go through a process that is going to take an hour long. During this time, there will be a tube that is inserted to the rectum. This is where the water will flow to go into the body in order to do its work along with any of the other nutrients that are going to be added in. After some time, there will be another tube that is added in that will work to allow all of the waste to go out of the body.

There are many different reasons why people would choose to go with this kind of therapy in order to make their lives healthier. The first one is for fecal incontinence. When this issue in present, there will need to be regular use of this kind of therapy is going to be used on a regular basis in order to clean out the lower intestine and make sure it is in the right working order. The next condition is going to be for ostomy care; if it is used for this, it will only be performed when absolutely necessary and there will need to be the constant supervision of a health care provider who is specialized in ostomy. Colonic spasm might be another reason that the therapy is used. A colonic spasm is going to be something that occurs when a colonoscopy has been performed and the intestines are not responding that well to it; when this happens, some colon hydrotherapy which uses warm water can help to relieve the spasms. These are the situations that have been studied and are usually the most accepted uses for colon hydrotherapy.

Of course, there are some other reasons that some people will choose to use colon hydrotherapy even if they do not have one of the conditions above and it is not approved by most doctors. Some people like the idea of cleaning out their intestines in order to help lose weight. They think that if they clear out the intestines that this will make them lighter while allowing the intestines to better absorb all of the nutrients they are taking in during their diet plan. Other people believe that doing this kind of hydrotherapy is going to help them to get rid of a lot of different illnesses that they might have. They think that the bacteria that is stuck in their body is going to make their immunity lower and so they might try to do some hydrotherapy in the hopes of making their bodies feel better to get rid of all the diseases and illnesses that they are dealing with.

There are some risks to worry about when it comes to using this kind of therapy though. While it does have some effective uses, it needs to be done in an effective way in order to avoid the adverse effects that can come with doing it. For example, if the practitioner who is working on this therapy with you is inserting too much of the water through this procedure, it is possible for you as the patient to suffer from an imbalance of electrolytes in the blood, fluid in the lungs, heart failure, and nausea. There might also be the risk of having a perforation of the bowels or an instance where the walls of your bowels will be broken due to the increase in fluid. If you do insist on doing this procedure, which is usually safe, just make sure that you are going to someone who is trained in this procedure so that you can avoid any of these issues and never attempt to do this on your own.

Before you go through a colon hydrotherapy, you should not only make sure that you are going to a professional who knows what they are doing, but also make sure that all of the equipment that they will use is sterile and has not been used without being cleaned since the last patient. When you take these measures, you are going to be able to greatly reduce the amount of risks that were listed above. Also, before you go through one of these therapies, talk to your regular doctor to see if this would actually benefit you or if you have some conditions that might be aggravated through this kind of therapy. There are some conditions such as tumors in rectum and the colon, internal hemorrhoids, Chron's disease, and diverticulitis, which can be worsened with the use of colon hydrotherapy. Sometimes it will be a better choice for you to just eat a healthy diet and go through a cleanse or detox in order to get the same kind of results.

Benefits of Colon Hydrotherapy

Now that you know a bit more about colon hydrotherapy, you might be interested in figuring out why you might want to go through this kind of therapy. It might not sound like the most comfortable procedure and the steps might make some people turn away from it even though there are a lot of benefits. Here are a few benefits that you will be able to get with the use of this therapy which can make it worth going through the procedure.

- Lose weight—many people choose to go through a colon hydrotherapy because they think it is an effective way for them to lose the weight that they want. They feel that it is going to clear up the intestines so that they are losing weight right away in that manner and then they look at it as a better way to absorb all of the good nutrients they are eating into the body, lowering the amount of hunger they are feeling. Whether the weight loss is actually happening due to the therapy is still unstudied, but many people swear that it was the thing that worked for them.

- Clear out intestines—some people just want to clear out the intestines in order to make themselves feeler. They might feel like they are lighter or healthier when the intestines or clear. Or they might just not like the idea that bacteria and old food is sitting in their bodies and so they will do this process to get rid of it. Of course, there has bene no evidence that there is a lot of bacteria and food sitting around in the intestines as the digestive system is really effective at getting rid of all this stuff, but that does not mean that if this process works for you to feel better that you should not try it out.

- Better absorption of nutrients in the body—the theory behind this kind of therapy is that it is able to help you to clear out all of the bad stuff that might be in your body. When this happens, it clears up the inner walls that are in the intestines so that they are free to do their job when it comes to absorbing the nutrients that are there. Whether you are doing this to lose weight or to just be healthier with the nutrients you take in, this therapy can be a great way to get it all done in an easy way.

- Prevent illnesses—some of those who decide to do this kind of therapy are going to be interested in it because they think it can prevent illnesses. This goes back to the idea that the bacteria that is stuck in the colon is reducing the immune system so it does not work and when you get rid of the bacteria, you are able to increase how effective the immunity is. When the colon is all cleared out, it can be possible that he body is going to be able to stay healthier and you will not have to deal with as many illnesses and diseases as you did before.

- Clearer head—it might be possible to get a clearer head after you are done with a colon hydrotherapy session. This is going to seem a little funny since the digestive system and the brain are not connected, but it makes sense when you remember that the nutrients are going to be able to get through easier. When the intestines are set up to absorb nutrients better, you are going to be able to get more of these tasty and healthy nutrients to the brain and it can do its job better. A cleaning up of the intestines may be just what that foggy brain needs in order to start feeling great again.

- Keep your energy up—those who have gone through this this therapy have found that their energy levels are up. They are going to feel like they are much lighter than before which can give them energy on its own. Many people who do this kind of therapy are going to use it before they start out on a new diet plan so the combination of clearing out the intestines and all of the good food they are eating is going to allow them to really get the energy levels they are looking for. Plus they are clearing out the intestines so that they are able to absorb the nutrients they are taking in much better.

- Prevent colon spasms—one of the approved methods of using this therapy that even doctors will recommend to their patients is to prevent colon spasms. It is not uncommon for someone to have these spasms after they have gone through a colonoscopy. The use of some warm water on the colon can help them to relax and to get the spasms to end. This is not going to necessarily be used as a cleanse, but can provide some relief to the person who going through the issue and can be performed in a hospital.

- Helps with detoxing—there are several different types of detoxing that are available and they can all be assisted with this therapy. The one that is usually prescribed with this therapy is to detox the body from a drug or substance. Some doctors or practitioners will recommend the therapy as a way to get the substance or drug out of the body in order to speed up the process. Some patients will choose to go with the therapy because they think it will help them to detox the body to help with weight loss in the long run.

As you can see, this is a fairly simple process that can be done for a wide variety of reasons. As long as you are following some of the suggestions for safety listed above, such as making sure to choose a licensed and trained professional and ensuring that the equipment has been sterilized before use, it is unlikely that you are going to run into any risks or trouble. When using this therapy, it will provide you with some of the great benefits that you saw above and can be a really effective way for you to improve your health in a wide variety of arenas.

Chapter 4: A Walk Through of a Session

Going to your first session of colon hydrotherapy can be a bit daunting. You want to make sure that you are going to be safe and secure when you go in, but the idea of what can go on in the session will scare some people away. Some of the worries might be from things you have read and others could come from friends and family who will tell you horror stories. Regardless of what you have heard about this therapy in the past, it is best to go through and learn the steps that actually occur before you go into a session, whether you are still considering the session or have already scheduled one.

Preparing for the Colon Hydrotherapy

There are a few things that you will be able to do in order to help prepare yourself for the session you will be undertaking. These are not necessarily requirements, but they can help you to relax down a bit as well as get the most out of the cleansing so that it works the way that you would like. It is up to you whether you would like to follow these suggestions or not, but they can help you out and make the session feel better.

7 to 10 days before the therapy

During this time, you need to make sure that you are eating the right kinds of foods. These are going to help you to get some better bowel movements and get the body all ready for the therapy to work at its best. If you are eating an unhealthy diet, the therapy might only be able to get some of the top layers since you have so much gunk in there. But if you are eating some good and healthy foods, such as doing the detoxes in previous chapters, you might be able to clear out the system a bit so that the therapy is able to concentrate more on some of the deeper gunk that needs to be taken care of. Some of the dietary suggestions that you can keep in mind for this time period include:

- Chew up the food completely. You will want it to be almost a liquid before you swallow for easier digestion.

- Drink at least half of the weight of your body in ounces. This means that if you weigh 160 pounds, you need to consume at least 10 glasses of water. If you are going to drink alcohol, soda, or coffee, you need to add another glass of the water for each one of these

- Avoid foods such as gluten, cereals, pizza, and pasta because they are going to get stuck up in the stomach and can make the therapy less effective.

- Increase the amount of fruits and vegetables that you consume. This is going to allow you to clear out the system a bit more and then you will have a better therapy session than before.

- Choose to eat some fish and chicken rather than pork and beef for better health overall.

You might also find that practicing some massage therapies on your stomach in the week or so before your therapy can help out. It will release some of the tension that you are feeling due to the thoughts about the therapy. Plus you are going to be able to learn the method that is going to work the best to calm you down and when the therapy is going on. You will then be able to use this on yourself or ask the therapist to help you out in order to remain calm and feel better when you get tense during the therapy.

2 hours before the session

A few hours before you go in for your session, you should make sure that you do not have a full stomach. It is often recommended that you avoid eating at least 2 hours before you go in to the session so that the stomach has time to empty out at least a little bit. If you feel that you are hungry or that your blood sugar feels a little low, it is fine to have a bit of a snack to keep you from getting stressed and hungry. Just make sure that you are avoiding anything that is too heavy and will get in the way of the therapy workings. You also must avoid any caffeine during your session. You can go a bit without caffeine and it is possible to have some after the session is over.

1 hour before the session

You should make sure that you are not drinking a lot of liquids before you have to go in to the session. It is often recommended that you stop drinking at least an hour before your session and then empty out the bladder right before starting. Of course you can drink something if you need before the session, but you will find that you are much more comfortable when you have a bladder that is not full when you begin the session.

15 minutes before the session

It is normal for you to feel a bit nervous before you go and get this session done. Some clients find that getting a message or doing some yoga or other relaxation technique allows them to be a little more relaxed. You might want to consider doing this before going in. If you do not have the time for this, you should find a way to relax and get rid of any stress that you might have for the day at least fifteen minutes before you go into your session. Try to be there a bit early so that you are able to sit down for at least a few minutes to calm down any nerves that you have. Compose any questions you have ahead of time in order to calm down before you go in. Remember that while this process might seem a bit strange, it is for your own health and learning how to be calm during it is a great idea.

How to dress

Many people are worried about the clothing that they will be wearing when it comes to this process. They are not sure what to do with it since this is not a procedure that a lot of people will have done. Some of the suggestions that you can follow to make sure that you are wearing the right clothing for the therapy includes:

- Wear something that is comfortable on top and that you can lay in for a bit. You will be disrobing from the waist down so this part is not going to be as important.

- It is often not recommended that you wear some long dresses. You will end up needing to hike them up and this can become uncomfortable on your stomach over the time of the therapy.

- Bring an extra shirt. In some rare occasions, there might be a bit of leakage during the session and your shirt might get a bit dirty. This is often not going to happen, but it is better to bring something along rather than have a dirty shirt

If you are able to follow a few of these hints when it comes to getting ready for the therapy, it is going to go a lot easier. Just remember to stay calm and relaxed and you will be surprised at how easy it can all be.

What to Expect at Your Session

The first thing you will do is go into the office. A therapist is going to greet you before asking if you would fill out a form about your past health and medical information. This will help them to determine if you will be eligible for this session or if you should be turned away because you have Chron's disease or another disorder that can be aggravated through the use of this therapy. The therapist is also going to take some time to discuss what you would like to get accomplished from the sessions and talk with you to ensure you do not have any questions before you begin. When ready, you will be taken to the proper room to begin the therapy. You should expect the first session to take around two hours but any of the ones you do after this will last a bit longer than an hour.

When you are in the room, you will learn about the proper way to be positioned by the colon therapist. They will help you to be on the table in the right way to make this process a little easier. They will also answer any of the questions you may have when it comes to the procedure before beginning. Then the therapist is going to go out of the room so that their client is able to have a moment of privacy to undress. You will just need to undress from the waist. Then you can get on the table in the way that the doctor showed to you and then you will insert the sterile rectal tube before covering with the towel they give you. This tube is only going to need to go a few inches into the rectum so it will not take too much, but if you are having difficulties with this, ask the therapist for some help.

Once you are all ready, the therapist is going to come back into the room in order to get things started, tell the monitor what it needs to do, and to help you out with anything else that you will need during this session. There are a variety of ways the therapist will be able to help you to relax if needed during the process including energy work, pressure point releasing, foot and hand reflexology, and abdominal massage.

After everything is in place and you are as comfortable as possible, some safe and temperature controlled water is going to flow through this rectal tube and straight into the colon. Any time you will feel like you need to release the water, this tube is going to move over to the side in the rectum so that the softened feces is allowed to just flow out. It is going to do this into a base that is connected to the rectal tube. There is also a system that is meant to release odor so that the area is not going to get all smelly.

You will stay in the room for the remainder of the therapy, which will usually last about an hour or so, letting this whole system continue on with a cleaning out of the colon in the process. The cleaning up process is going to be easy for you since it has already been drained out while you are going through the therapy. After each of the sessions, the therapist is going to check and make sure the patient is doing well and then you can be set up to get another one done in the future if you would like and depending on the reasons that you are using this therapy.

When the client is done, the therapist and their office will need to thoroughly clean and then disinfect the tools that were used and then it will be all ready to use again on the next client. This is all there is to the therapy. It is pretty easy and straightforward and is not as worrisome as many people would think. Other than the initial shock of getting the tubes placed in, you will basically just let the therapy happen, with a little help of relaxation techniques if needed to keep calm during the session to make it work out much better.

Conclusion

When you are worried about the digestive system not working the way that it should and you want to get it back up and running, a colon hydrotherapy might be the best choice for you. Of course, this therapy is only going to be able to do so much and a healthy detox and diet, like those described in this book are often some great choices to have along with the hydrotherapy if you choose to go down this road. While the therapy might seem like it is a bit strange to those who are new to it, there are so many health and life benefits of going with it, that it really makes sense to try it out.

This guidebook is meant to help you to understand more about your digestive system and the use of colon hydrotherapy in order to keep the digestive system working at its very best. You will learn that this therapy is not all that scary and that it can really do wonders for your whole body. Take a look through this book and see how great you can look and feel with the help of the right tools.

About the Author

I am Marina, the owner of Scottsdale Hydrotherapy. It took me 17 years of trial and error to overcome my digestive and gut issues.

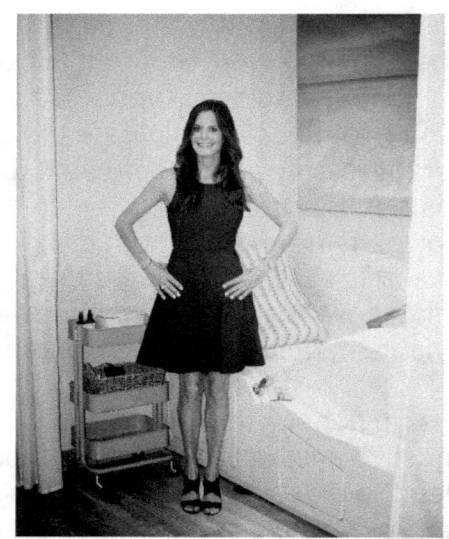

Through colon hydrotherapy and clean eating, I not only found the relief I was seeking but also a boost in health and Energy. The restorative impact of detoxifying my body through colon irrigation was exactly what I needed.

With Scottsdale Hydrotherapy I am able to share this healing with others, help them take charge, and enhance their own health.

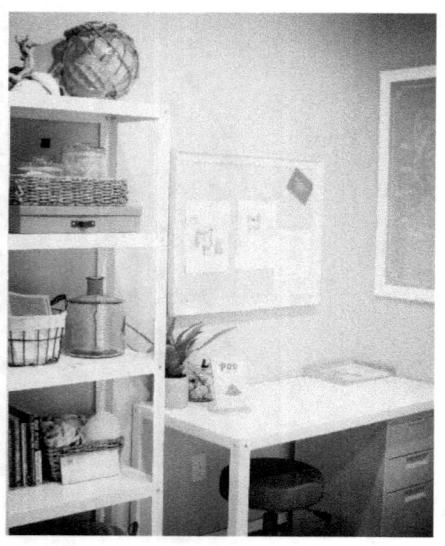

At Scottsdale Hydrotherapy we look at your symptoms while addressing your body as a whole.

We see a wide range of clients at our practice. Many have been getting colonics regularly (one to four times per month) for years, others come to us on the advice of their medical professionals, and as awareness about the benefits of colon hydrotherapy grows we are seeing more and more first timers.

There are strict FDA guidelines that Scottsdale Hydrotherapy must follow to ensure your safety. We use top of the line FDA approved equipment. Our North Scottsdale office prides itself on being professional, private and discrete.

www.ingramcontent.com/pod-product-compliance
Lightning Source LLC
Chambersburg PA
CBHW060445290526
45793CB00002B/584